YOUR KNOWLEDGE HAS VALUE

- We will publish your bachelor's and master's thesis, essays and papers

- Your own eBook and book - sold worldwide in all relevant shops

- Earn money with each sale

Upload your text at www.GRIN.com
and publish for free

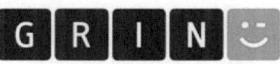

Bibliographic information published by the German National Library

The German National Library lists this publication in the National Bibliography; detailed bibliographic data are available on the Internet at http://dnb.dnb.de .

This book is copyright material and must not be copied, reproduced, transferred, distributed, leased, licensed or publicly performed or used in any way except as specifically permitted in writing by the publishers, as allowed under the terms and conditions under which it was purchased or as strictly permitted by applicable copyright law. Any unauthorized distribution or use of this text may be a direct infringement of the author s and publisher s rights and those responsible may be liable in law accordingly.

Imprint:

Copyright © 2018 GRIN Verlag, Open Publishing GmbH
Print and binding: Books on Demand GmbH, Norderstedt Germany
ISBN: 9783668623019

This book at GRIN:

https://www.grin.com/document/388524

Patrick Kimuyu

Microbial Flora Changes during UHT Pasteurization of Milk

GRIN - Your knowledge has value

Since its foundation in 1998, GRIN has specialized in publishing academic texts by students, college teachers and other academics as e-book and printed book. The website www.grin.com is an ideal platform for presenting term papers, final papers, scientific essays, dissertations and specialist books.

Visit us on the internet:

http://www.grin.com/

http://www.facebook.com/grincom

http://www.twitter.com/grin_com

Content

Introduction 2

Control of Contamination during Preparation Stage 2

Transfer of Raw Milk to Heat Exchangers 3

Decontamination at 63^0C to 72^0C 3

Decontamination at 73^0C to 150^0C 4

Control of Contamination during Pre-packaging Stage 5

Control of Contamination during Packaging 5

Hermetic Sealing 6

Conclusion 6

References 7

Introduction

In the food production industry, food spoilage by microorganisms poses an immense challenge to food sustainability and health safety. Most of the preservation methods are aimed at destroying the microbial populations that are present in the raw materials, preventing contamination, improving the texture of the manufactured food products, and creating desired flavours (Walstra 2013). For instance, Ultra-High Temperature pasteurization, commonly referred to as UHT pasteurization is a preservation method that is carried out to decontaminate raw food products. This preservation method is used predominantly in milk processing, unlike its alternative processing method, High Temperature/Short-Time pasteurization which is used to process an array of raw food materials. In most cases, raw milk is usually contaminated with bacteria, moulds and yeast microbes. However, bacteria constitute the greatest percentage of microbial populations in raw milk based on studies which have found different pathogenic bacteria in raw milk, especially *L. monocytogenes*, *Salmonella spp*, *Campylobacter spp* and *E. coli* (Tremonte et al. 2014). Therefore, this article provides a comprehensive discussion on how the microbial flora changes during Ultra-High Temperature pasteurization.

Control of Contamination during Preparation Stage

Foremost, UHT pasteurization involves the preparation of raw milk prior to the actual pasteurization process. In most cases, *Mycobacterium spp* are usually present in raw milk from cows because cattle serve as hosts for these mycobacteria especially *M. bovis* which has been the concern in international trade of most animal products (Franco et al. 2013). However, most of the bacteria which are involved in milk spoilage are from the environment. Some of the main sources of contamination of milk during UHT pasteurization, as well as other milk processing methods are the udder and hygiene (Cempírková 2007). During milking, milk is likely to become contaminated within the teat canal epithelium. Teat canal and the udder are usually inhabited by an array of normal skin microflora comprising of streptococci and *micrococci* species (Hantsis-Zacharov & Halpern 2007). Therefore, contamination of milk with these bacteria is controlled through the adoption of safe milking practices such as washing of the udder before milking.

Transfer of Raw Milk to Heat Exchangers

The second step in milk preparation during UHT pasteurization involves the transfer of milk from the milking plant to the preservation apparatus. In most cases, milk contamination occurs during this step due to poor handling of raw milk. Evidence shows that vessels such as milk cans which are used to hold milk before processing contain microorganisms. Some of the bacteria that are commonly found on the surfaces of milk cans include *Brucella spp*, *Enterobacter* and *Clostridium spp* (Scott 2008). Therefore, milk handling prior to the process of pasteurization determines the degree of raw milk contamination. In order to minimize contamination at this stage, high standards of hygiene are recommended to ensure raw milk is not contaminated through handling. One of the most appropriate control measures is disinfecting milk holding vessels to destroy biofilms which may be present in the equipments (Scott 2008).

However, any contamination during the steps before UHT pasteurization is controlled during the actual preservation in heat exchangers which eliminate all microorganisms in raw milk, as well as destroying bacteria toxins and spores. In UHT pasteurization, milk is heated to 138^0 to 150^0 C (280^0 to 302^0 F) for 1 to 2 seconds. As a result, temperature changes during the heating process coincide with changes in the microbial flora in raw milk. Ordinarily, most bacteria in raw milk exhibit optimal activity between 20^0 C and 30^0 C. However, it is worth noting that bacteria can ferment milk at low temperatures, even below 7^0 C as it has been observed with psychrotrophic bacteria (Munsch-Alatossava & Alatossava 2006).

Decontamination at 63°C to 72°C

Once milk is placed in heat exchangers for UHT pasteurization, temperatures are raised over time to reach the ideal temperature for destroying all microbial flora including microbial proteins such toxins. As the temperature increases from 30^0 C, the optimal temperate upon which bacteria growth occurs to 63^0 C, most non-spore-forming bacteria are eliminated through destruction by heat. In practice, temperatures between 63^0 C and 72^0 C have been found to be ideal in destroying microbial flora in milk (Scott 2008). This is the concept applied in other pasteurization techniques used in processing milk in which milk is heated to 63^0 C to 72^0 C for some time, in order to destroy bacteria. Therefore, raising temperature up to 72^0 C ensures all non-sporeforming bacteria are destroyed. Bacteria species which are destroyed by temperatures include *Pseudomonas spp*, *Pantoea spp*, *Leuconostoc mesenteroides*, *Acinebacter spp*, *Lactococcus spp*, *Enterobacter spp*, and *Psychrobacter spp*. Other non-sporeforming bacteria species which are destroyed by heat increase to 72^0 C are *Kurthia gibsonii* and *Exiguobacterum spp* (Anzueto 2014). It is also worth noting that all bacteria species of bovine origin such as *Mycobacterium tuberculosis* and *Brucella spp* are destroyed at this temperature range.

Non-sporeforming bacteria remaining are usually destroyed as the heat exchanger temperatures rise to 100^0 C. It is also worth noting that some spore-forming bacteria species are destroyed at pasteurization temperatures below 100^0 C. However, most spore-forming bacteria have been found to withstand high temperatures, and this is attributable to their adaptive traits, primarily the formation of heat-resistant spores. Therefore, almost all heat-resistant bacteria in milk are destroyed by the time temperatures within the heat exchangers increase to 138^0 C. In practice, UHT pasteurization occurs by heating milk between 138^0 C and 150^0 C for 1 to 2 seconds. This temperature is ideal for destroying all bacteria spores which remain after active cells are destroyed at lower temperatures during the heat treatment process. Therefore, bacteria spores which are present in milk are destroyed at this level. Microbial floras which are destroyed at this step include *Bacillus spp*, *Clostridium botulinum*, *Brevibacillus spp*, *Paenisporosarcna*, *Paenibacillus spp*, and *Lysinibacillus spp*. In most cases, *Bacillus spp* including *Bacillus licheniformis*, *Bacillus aerophilus*, *Bacillus safensis*, and *Bacillus subtilis* are known to be the most heat-resistant bacteria species causing milk spoilage (Anzueto 2014).

Decontamination at 73ºC to 150ºC

Ideally, increasing the temperatures above 72^0 C up to 15^0C eliminates heat-resistant microbial floras in their order of heat susceptibility. For instance, all spore-forming microbial floras are eliminated under temperatures between 72^0 C and 120^0 C including *Bacillus cereas* (Scott 2008). Above the temperature of 120^0 C, only five bacteria species exist in milk during UHT pasteurization. These microbial populations include *Bacillus licheniformis*, *Brevibacillus borstelensis*, *Bacillus subtilis*, *Paenibacillus*, and *Aneurinibacillus* (Scheldeman et al. 2005). Therefore, temperatures for UHT pasteurization (138^0 C to 150^0 C) ensures all heat-resistant bacteria are destroyed. In addition, this temperature destroys microbial toxins that may contribute to food spoilage. For instance, microbial toxins such as *Botulinum* neurotoxin are inactivated by heating milk at 72^0 C and beyond (Weingart et al. 2010). As such, the milk is said to be sterile. Therefore, UHT pasteurization leads to the production of sterile milk whose shelf-life is extended (Scott 2008). Ordinarily, UHT pasteurized milk stays in the shelves for up to 90 days without getting spoiled by microorganisms. However, sterility of UHT pasteurized milk depends on several factors which precede the heat treatment process.

Control of Contamination during Pre-packaging Stage
In some circumstances, UHT pasteurized milk gets contaminated during packaging. Putrefying bacteria, as well as pathogenic bacteria can be reintroduced in heat treated milk due to post-treatment processing. For instance, holding pre-heated milk unpackaged in septic containers increases the risk of contamination with microorganisms (Scott 2008). It is relatively easy for bacteria, yeast and moulds to find their way into the pasteurized milk. In order to minimize contamination after the heating process, milk should be packaged within 3 minutes. Holding milk for more than 3 minutes increases the risk of contamination leading to milk spoilage before the intended shelf-life.

Control of Contamination during Packaging
Another entry of contaminating bacteria after UHT pasteurization is the packaging process. In some circumstances, pasteurized milk gets contaminated during packaging. According to good industrial dairy products processing practices, UHT pasteurized milk should be packaged in sterile containers to prevent microbial contamination. Sterilization of containers including bottles and cans is usually done through different sterilization methods. For instance, autoclaving is applied in sterilizing milk packaging materials. On the other hand, irradiation with UV rays is, in most cases, used to sterilize containers for dairy products. Another useful method of sterilization of containers used in packaging dairy products is dry hot-air, a sterilization technique which is also used in meat canning (Scott 2008). Therefore, the use of sterile packaging containers serves as a significant control measure that prevents the contamination of UHT pasteurized end products.

Hermetic Sealing

In addition, packaging UHT pasteurized milk should be accompanied by appropriate sealing of the containers. In practice, heat-treated milk should be packaged in airtight containers, a practice referred to as hermetic sealing. Hermetic sealing is usually done to prevent entry of microorganisms during milk storage. In most cases, UHT pasteurized milk gets spoiled before its shelf-life lapses owing to improper sealing of containers. For instance, milk packaged in containers with loose seals is likely to allow entry for microorganisms leading to fast spoilage. In order to prevent milk contamination after packaging, milk containers should be tightly-sealed to ensure that damage to the seal does not occur during transportation or storage. UHT pasteurization of milk is usually characterized by a more stringent packaging compared to other pasteurization techniques such as ultra-pasteurization and flash pasteurization. This is the reason why UHT pasteurized milk does not require refrigeration to extent its shelf-life.in addition, UHT pasteurized milk can stay in the shelves for as long as 90 days (Scott 2008). As such, UHT pasteurization preserves milk for the longest period compared to all other preservation methods.

Conclusion

Conclusively, food preservation is considered as the most appropriate way of controlling food spoilage. This approach is ideal in achieving food sustainability through minimizing spoilage of agricultural food products. Therefore, food preservation or processing is a crucial aspect in food manufacturing. This is so because; it extends the shelf-life of the end products compared to raw materials. In milk processing, raw milk petrify within hours due to the fermentation activity of microorganisms, primarily bacteria, moulds and yeast. Evidence shows that milk contains microbial contaminants long before it is milked from the cow. This phenomenon is attributable to the presence of normal microbial flora which are found in teats canal epithelium and the udder. In addition, milk may be contaminated with pathogenic microorganisms such as *Mycobacterium tuberculosis* and *Brucella spp* (Hantsis-Zacharov & Halpern 2007). Therefore, UHT pasteurization of milk decontaminates milk hence increasing its shelf-life, as well as reducing exposure of humans to pathogenic bacteria and toxic proteins. During the entire process of UHT pasteurization ranging from pre-heating preparations to packaging, microbial profile changes gradually until the end product is produced. Control of contamination with microorganisms begins with hygienic handling of raw milk. The second step in decontaminating milk is the heat treatment during UHT pasteurization in which milk is heated up to 150^0 C. Ordinarily, raising the temperature beyond 63^0 C ensures microorganisms, primarily bacteria are destroyed. At 72^0 C, most microbial populations present in raw milk are already destroyed (Scott 2008). However, heat-resistant spore-forming bacteria may withstand temperatures as high as 138^0 C. Therefore, heating milk at 138^0 C to 150^0 C ensures that all vegetative spores, as well as microbial toxins are destroyed.

References

Anzueto, ME 2014, *Tracking heat-resistant, sporeforming bacteria in the milk chain: a farm to table approach*, M.Sc Thesis, University of Nebraska, viewed 10 Jan 2018, http://digitalcommons.unl.edu/cgi/viewcontent.cgi?article=1045&context=foodscidiss

Cempírková, R 2007, Contamination of cow's raw milk by psychrotrophic and mesophilic microflora in relation to selected factors, *Czech J. Anim. Sci.*, vol. 52 no. 11, pp. 387–393.

Franco, J, Paes, AC, Ribeiro, MG, Pantoja, JC, Santos, AC, Miyata, M, Leite, CQ, Motta, RG, & Listoni, FJ 2013, Occurrence of mycobacteria in bovine milk samples from both individual and collective bulk tanks at farms and informal markets in the southeast region of Sao Paulo, Brazil, *BMC Veterinary Research* vol. 9, pp. 85.

Hantsis-Zacharov, E & Halpern, M 2007, Culturable psychrotrophic bacterial communities in raw milk and their proteolytic and lipolytic traits, *Applied and Environmental Microbiology* vol. 73, pp. 7162-7168.

Munsch-Alatossava, P & Alatossava, T 2006, Phenotypic characterization of raw milk-associated psychrotrophic bacteria, *Microbiological Research*, vol. 161 no. 4, pp. 334–346.

Scheldeman, P, Pil, A, Herman, L, De Vos, P & Heyndrick, M 2005, Incidence and diversity of potentially highly heat-resistant spores isolated at dairy farms, *Applied Environmental Microbiology* vol. 71 no. 3, pp. 1480-1494.

Scott, DL 2008, *UHT processing and aseptic filling of dairy foods*, PHD Thesis, Kansas State University, viewed 22 June 2015, < http://krex.k-state.edu/dspace/bitstream/handle/2097/970/DavidScott2008.pdf?sequence=1 >

Tremonte, P, Tipaldi, L, Succi, M, Pannella. G, Falasca, L, Capilongo, V, Coppola, R, & Sorrentino, E 2014, Raw milk from vending machines: Effects of boiling, microwave treatment, and refrigeration on microbiological quality, *Journal of Dairy Science* vol. 97 no. 6, pp. 3314–3320.

Walstra, P 2013, *Dairy technology: principles of milk properties and processes*, CRC Press, Boca Raton.

Weingart, OG, Schreiber, T, Mascher, C, Pauly, D, Dorner, MB, Berger, TF, Egger, C, Gessler, F, Loessner, MJ, Avondet, M & Dorner, BG 2010, The Case of Botulinum Toxin in Milk: Experimental Data, *Appl Environ Microbiol.*, vol. 76 no. 10, pp. 3293–3300.

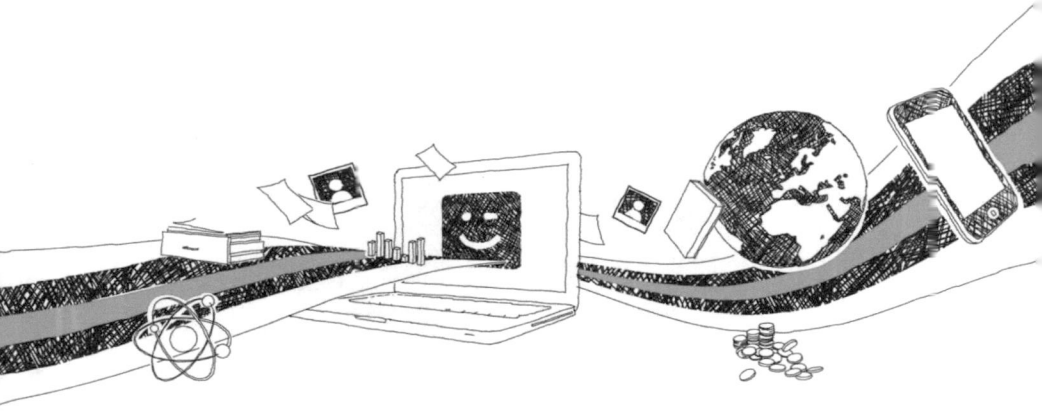